Pegan Diet Cookbook

100% VEGAN

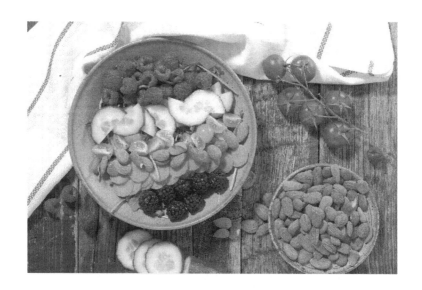

Your Personalized Guide to Losing Weight, Reducing Inflammation, and Feeling Amazing

By Karen Greenvang

Copyright ©Karen Greenvang 2016

1

D1565368

All information in this book has been carefully researched and checked for factual accuracy. However, the author and publishers make no warranty, expressed or implied, that the information contained herein is appropriate for every individual, situation or purpose, and assume no responsibility for errors or omission. The reader assumes the risk and full responsibility for all actions, and the author will not be held liable for any loss or damage, whether consequential, incidental, and special or otherwise, that may result from the information presented in this publication.

All cooking is an experiment in a sense, and many people come to the same or similar recipe over time. All recipes in this book have been derived from author's personal experience. Should any bear a close resemblance to those used elsewhere, that is purely coincidental.

Table of Contents

Introduction- Pegan Recipes

In the last few years the health and diet scene has witnessed a large shift towards the idea of going back to basics in the form of the caveman or Paleo diet. This diet centers around the concept of eating only foods that our hunter-gatherer ancestors would have had access to and therefore eliminates all processed foods and focuses on whole foods in their simplest form.

The Pegan diet is where the concepts of vegan and paleo meet and has many health benefits that will help you sustain a healthy lifestyle based around a nutritionally sound way of eating. The pegan diet consists of mainly fruits, vegetables, nuts, seeds, avocados, olives, and coconut. Grains, legumes and soy products are excluded as they all require some form of processing. Any form of refined sugars is also excluded.

There are many benefits to a pegan diet that include a low glycemic load as refined carbohydrates of any kind are excluded. The high density of fresh fruits and vegetables provide essential vitamins, minerals and fibre. The nuts, seeds, avocados, olives and coconut provide heart healthy, good quality fats. One would think that the pegan diet would be lacking in protein, but you will be getting a sufficient amount of this essential dietary component from the nuts which form a part of most of the recipes. Possibly the most notable benefit of the pegan diet is that by eliminating processed foods you are not exposing yourself to unhealthy chemical additives and preservatives. By sticking to organically grown produce as much as possible you are reducing your exposure to pesticides, antibiotics and hormones that are used in the commercial farming processes.

1951's Vegan Society definition of veganism: "Veganism is the doctrine that humans should live without exploiting animals."

Vegan cuisine is based on the exclusion of all animal products, including meat, eggs, dairy, honey, gelatin etc. Many people are aware of the abuse inflicted on animals and would like to experiment with a healthier diet, that is environmentally conscious and cautious and respectful of animals. Often people are discouraged by the lack of recipes or tools to achieve it. This book attempts to address this problem and also to supplement the needs of long-time vegans who would like to add a variety of textures and looks to their dishes while keeping it grain-free and soy free.

So, to make it simple, the recipes contained in this book are both vegan-friendly and paleo friendly. They are also naturally gluten-free.

This book is an excellent choice for:

-vegans and vegetarians

-anyone interested in a plant-based lifestyle

-anyone wishing to add more fresh fruits and vegetables into their diets

-paleo diet followers who would like to explore more of a gatherer's side of this diet

-gluten-free diet followers

-anyone wishing to eat more alkaline and raw to restore natural energy

-low carb diet followers

The recipes in this book will give you inspiration and an abundance of ideas to plan healthy, satisfying and nutritious meals that all fit within pegan way of eating. There are three sections, each focusing on the three main meals within your day; breakfast, lunch and dinner. There is also a smoothie section. Many of these recipes are based on raw foods, but some do require some cooking. Both styles are allowed on the pegan diet, it's up to you if you want to eat fully raw or just part time raw.

The beauty of these recipes is that they create meals that are very easy to have on the go since they consist of such simple and basic ingredients.

If you feel sick and tired of feeling sick and tired and wish to restore energy and zest for life, try to eat a pegan diet for at least a week. At the same time, remember to drink plenty of water and eliminate caffeine and sugar drinks. Even if you eat this way 80% of the time, you will still be able to energize yourself. Personally, I eat a fully vegan diet as this is my personal choice. My vegan diet is balanced, but I like to focus on pegan recipes or raw food recipes whenever I need more energy- I usually go pegan (grain free, no legumes, no process foods and I eat mostly raw or only slightly cooked pegan style recipes) for a week or two, whenever my body needs it. Or, I simply try to add more raw, unprocessed foods into my diet. These are both vegan (no animal products) and paleo-gatherer (no grains, no soy, no legumes, no gluten) friendly.

This is the best of the 2 worlds!

By eating more fresh vegetables and fruits you alkalize the heck out of yourself.

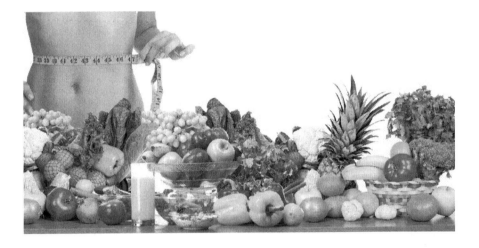

You see, our blood's optimal pH should be 7.35- which is slightly alkaline. By adding more alkaline foods (=fresh fruits and veggies that are naturally rich in vitamins and minerals) we help our body regulate its optimal blood pH. If we fail to do so and we eat processed foods that are acid-forming, we torture our body with incredible stress. If we constantly eat foods that are acid-forming, we eventually get sick as out body can no longer regulate its pH for us. The pegan diet is naturally alkaline-forming and helps us restore energy without overcomplicated pH discussions.

Just eat more fresh fruits and veggies, it's as simple as that. This rule is compatible with all the diets- vegan, vegetarian, paleo, low carb, high carb, gluten free + many more.

Free Complimentary eBook

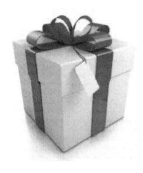 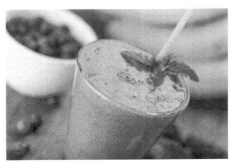

Before we dive into the recipes, I would like to offer you a free, complimentary recipe eBook with delicious vegan superfood smoothies. **Download link:**

www.bitly.com/karenfreegift

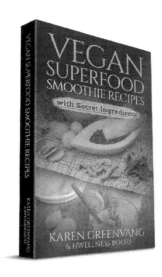

Breakfasts

As we all know breakfast is the most important meal of the day as it breaks the fast of sleeping and kick starts your metabolism allowing your body to adequately process and absorb all the foods, energy and nutrients that you consume throughout the day. A breakfast that is nutrient dense and high in fibre is the best way to start your day. The recipes in this section will provide you with a variety of essential vitamins, minerals and healthy fats that will satisfy that early morning hunger and keep you going right on to your mid-morning snack.

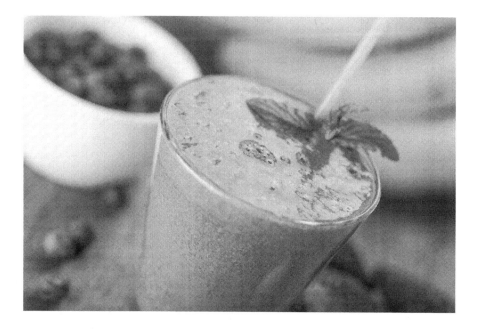

Tropical Breakfast with Papaya, Pineapple, Brazil nuts and Coconut Shavings

Both papaya and pineapple are very high in vitamin C, antioxidants and the essential minerals potassium, copper and magnesium. Pineapples are known for their anti-inflammatory benefits as well as their ability to help prevent macular degeneration. Brazil nuts are high in selenium which an essential trace mineral that is necessary for cognitive function, making these nuts a great breakfast choice. Together with the Brazil nuts, the coconut shavings not only add a complimentary flavor, but they also bring along their healthy fat content. Serve with a glass of chilled coconut milk and you have a well-rounded breakfast.

Serves One:

Ingredients:

- ½ Cup (125ml) Diced Fresh Papaya

- ½ Cup (125ml) Diced Fresh Pineapple

- 1 Tablespoon (15ml) Raw Brazil nuts, roughly chopped

- 1 Tablespoon (15ml) Raw Coconut Shavings

- 1 Cup (250ml) Coconut Milk (to serve)

Instructions:

1. In a serving bowl mix the diced papaya and pineapple together

2. Sprinkle the chopped Brazil nuts and coconut shavings over the top

3. Serve with the chilled coconut milk as a drink

Berry Delicious Breakfast with Almonds

Berries are very high in antioxidants and immune-boosting properties. The mix of berries in this recipe will provide you with a good variety of flavor, and essential minerals. The almonds bring along the protein and essential fats, as well as their high content of essential minerals. This dish can also be served with a glass of chilled coconut milk to add a little extra essential fat content.

Serves One:

Ingredients:

- ¼ Cup (60ml) Fresh strawberries, chopped

- ¼ Cup (60ml) Fresh raspberries, whole

- ¼ Cup (60ml) Fresh blueberries, whole

- ¼ Cup (60ml) Fresh gooseberries, whole

- ¼ Cup (60ml) Fresh cherries, pitted and halved

- ¼ Cup (60ml) Fresh mulberries, whole

- ¼ Cup (60ml) Raw almonds, roughly chopped

- 1 Cup (250ml) Chilled coconut milk, for serving

Instructions:

1. Mix all the berries together in a serving bowl

2. Sprinkle the roughly chopped almonds over the berries

3. Serve with the chilled coconut milk as a drink

Banana, Pecan nut and Date Breakfast

Bananas are high in potassium and energy making them a very good breakfast choice as they provide a healthy dose of nutrient rich carbohydrate. Pecan nuts are known for their protein content as well as their ability to lower bad cholesterol. Dates are great source of the essential minerals iron, calcium, magnesium, zinc; and are very high in fibre.

Serves One:

Ingredients:

- 1 large banana, sliced

- 1 Tablespoon (15ml) Raw pecan nuts, roughly chopped

- ¼ Cup (60ml) Dates, roughly chopped

- 1 Cup (250ml) Chilled coconut milk, for serving

Instructions:

- Place the sliced banana and dates in a serving bowl

- Sprinkle the chopped pecan nuts over the banana and dates

- Serve with the chilled coconut milk as a drink

- It is important to eat this breakfast soon after preparation as the banana will begin to brown if exposed to air for too long.

Citrus Medley Breakfast with Seeds

Citrus fruits are known for their high vitamin C and antioxidant properties, they are also great for boosting the immune system. The orange rind is high in flavanoids and essential minerals, making it worth including; it also adds a little zest to the overall flavor. Seeds are high in healthy omega 3 fats and provide a good source of energy.

Serve One:

Ingredients:

- 1 medium sized orange

- 1 medium sized grapefruit

- 1 Tablespoon (15ml) Raw seed mix

- Zest of the orange, grated

Instructions:

1. Using an orange-zester grate the orange peel into a bowl

2. Peel off the remaining pith of the orange and divide it into segments, place it in a serving bowl

3. Peel the grapefruit, divide it into segments and add it to the serving bowl with the orange

4. Sprinkle the raw seeds over the grapefruit and orange

5. Sprinkle the orange zest over the grapefruit, orange and seed mix

6. Toss together and serve

Apple, Pear and Cashew Nut Breakfast

Apples are very rich in essential anti-oxidants and are believed to help fight cancer; being a fruit that is known for its low glycemic index it is a great option for breakfast. Pears are known to be one of the fruits that are highest in fibre which also makes them a great choice for an energy sustaining breakfast. Cashew nuts provide protein, essential minerals and healthy fats.

Serves One:

Ingredients:

- 1 small red apple

- 1 small green apple

- 1 small green pear

- 1 small brown (also known as Asian) pear

- 1 Tablespoon (15ml) Raw cashew nuts, roughly chopped

Instructions:

1. Core the apples, slice them.

2. Place the apples in a serving bowl

3. Slice the pears and add them to the bowl with the apples

4. Sprinkle the chopped cashew nuts over the bowl with the pears and apples

5. It is important to eat this breakfast soon after preparation as the apples and pears will go brown with exposure to air, once they have been sliced.

Banana Porridge with Grapes and Pistachios

This recipe shows how one can be creative with the concept of a caveman plant based diet. By mashing the banana with the coconut milk in order to create a porridge-like consistency you are still able to have the comforting feel of a bowl of porridge without sacrificing your intent to exclude grains from your diet. The grapes are high in essential minerals and vitamin C, and add both color and extra sweetness to the overall dish. Pistachios are high in protein, essential fats and fibre.

Serves One:

Ingredients:

- 1 medium sized banana

- ¼ Cup (60ml) Coconut milk

- ¼ Cup (60ml) White grapes, halved

- ¼ Cup (60ml) Red grapes, halved

- 1 Tablespoon (15ml) Raw pistachio nuts, roughly chopped

- 1 Tablespoon (15ml) Coconut shavings

Instructions;

- In a serving bowl, mash the banana with the coconut milk to form a porridge consistency

- Add the grapes to the banana porridge and mix together

- Sprinkle the chopped pistachio nuts and coconut shavings over the banana porridge and serve

- If you would like to make this breakfast even more comforting, you could warm the coconut milk before adding it to the banana for mashing.

Banana Porridge with Berries and Almonds

This recipe is a variation on the previous banana porridge recipe that includes berries and almonds, combining the great energy source of the banana with the high anti-oxidant levels of the berries. The almonds bring some protein crunch to this comforting breakfast.

Serves One

Ingredients:

- 1 medium sized banana

- ¼ Cup (60ml) Coconut milk

- ¼ Cup (60ml) Fresh strawberries, chopped

- ¼ Cup (60ml) Fresh raspberries, whole

- ¼ Cup (60ml) Fresh blueberries, whole

- 1 Tablespoon (15ml) Raw almonds, roughly chopped

- 1 Tablespoon (15ml) Coconut shavings

Instructions:

1. In a serving bowl, mash the banana with the coconut milk to form a porridge consistency

2. Add the berries to the banana porridge and mix together

3. Sprinkle the almonds and coconut shavings over the banana porridge and serve

4. If you would like to make this breakfast even more comforting, you could warm the coconut milk before adding it to the banana for mashing.

Apple Porridge with Dates and Hazel Nuts

This recipe is another way in which you can get creative with the caveman concept, but it does require some cooking in order to get the apple to a porridge consistency. Given the low glycemic and high fibre properties of apples, along with the protein provided by the hazel nuts, this is a great breakfast option for sustained energy, and is very comforting as it can be served warm.

Serves One:

Ingredients:

- 1 small red apple, cored and chopped

- 1 small green apple, cored and chopped

- ¼ Cup (60ml) Dates, chopped

- 1 Tablespoon (15ml) Raw hazel nuts, roughly chopped

- 1 Cup (250ml) Coconut milk

- 1 Tablespoon (15ml) Coconut shavings

Instructions:

1. Place the chopped apple and the coconut milk in a saucepan

2. Bring the saucepan to the boil and then reduce to a low heat and allow to simmer until the apples are thoroughly cooked and soft

3. Once the apples have cooked and are very soft, remove the saucepan from the heat and mash up the apples to form a porridge-like consistency

4. If you are choosing to serve this breakfast warm, then place the apples in a serving bowl immediately. If you would prefer to serve this breakfast cold, then you will need to allow the apples to cool completely before placing them in a serving bowl.

5. Add the dates and chopped hazel nuts to the apple porridge

6. Sprinkle the coconut shavings over the top of the porridge and serve

Apple Porridge with Fresh Cherries and Brazil Nuts

This recipe is a variation on the previous apple porridge combination that includes fresh cherries which are known for their high anti-oxidant and cancer fighting properties.

Serves One:

Ingredients:

- 1 small red apple, cored and chopped

- 1 small green apple, cored and chopped

- ½ Cup (125ml) fresh cherries, pitted and halved

- 1 Cup (250ml) Coconut milk

- 1 Tablespoon (15ml) Raw Brazil nuts, roughly chopped

- 1 Tablespoon (15ml) Coconut shavings

Instructions:

1. Place the chopped apple and the coconut milk in a saucepan

2. Bring the saucepan to the boil and then reduce to a low heat and allow to simmer until the apples are thoroughly cooked and soft

3. Once the apples have cooked and are very soft, remove the saucepan from the heat and mash up the apples to form a porridge-like consistency

4. If you are choosing to serve this breakfast warm, then place the apples in a serving bowl immediately. If you would prefer to serve this breakfast cold, then you will need to allow the apples to cool completely before placing them in a serving bowl.

5. Add the cherries and chopped Brazil nuts to the apple porridge

6. Sprinkle the coconut shavings over the top of the porridge and serve

Cherry Tomatoes with Mushrooms, Avocado, Pistachios and Rosemary

Breakfast time always has room for something savory and this recipe is a great option for those days when that's what your mood calls for. Tomatocs are high in vitamin C, anti-oxidants and essential minerals. Mushrooms are a good source of selenium and vitamin D. Avocados are high in potassium and essential fats. This is another of those breakfast recipes that is best cooked as the process of doing so helps release the flavors of the mushrooms.

Serves One:

Ingredients:

- ½ Cup (125ml) Cherry tomatoes, halved

- ¼ Cup (60ml) White button mushrooms

- ¼ Cup (60ml) Black mushrooms

- 1 Teaspoon (5ml) fresh garlic, finely chopped

- 1 Teaspoon (5ml) fresh rosemary

- 1 ripe avocado, halved and pitted

- 1 Tablespoon (15ml) Extra Virgin Olive oil

- 1 Tablespoon (15ml) Raw pistachio nuts, roughly chopped

Instructions:

1. Heat the olive oil in a saucepan

2. Add the garlic and rosemary, fry until the garlic has softened

3. Add the mushrooms and turn the heat down to a medium one, cover the saucepan with its lid and allow the mushrooms to reduce

4. Once the mushrooms have started boiling in their own water, remove the lid from the saucepan and allow all the liquid to cook off the mushrooms

5. Once the mushrooms begin to brown, add the tomatoes and cook at a medium/high heat until both the mushrooms and tomatoes have browned and cooked through

6. Place the avocado halves on a plate and fill each half with the mushroom and tomato mixture

7. Sprinkle the chopped pistachios over the stuffed avocado halves and serve

Lunches

Lunchtime is a great time of the day because it gives us a necessary break to refuel our bodies for the afternoon stretch to dinner time. The recipes in this section comprise mainly of salads that arc easy to prepare and take with you to work or on a picnic. They include a variety of vegetables, fresh herbs, healthy fats and some fruits; all ingredients that will help sustain your energy throughout the afternoon.

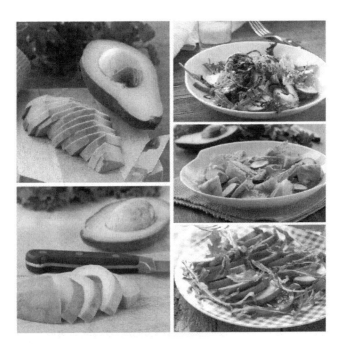

Fresh Coriander Salad with Seeds and Cashew Nuts

Coriander is a great source of essential minerals and dietary fibre. The selection of raw vegetables that this salad includes also provides a healthy dose of vitamins, minerals and fibre. The seeds add a healthy dose of fats and the cashew nuts provide the protein, as well as a little extra healthy fat.

Serves One:

Ingredients:

- 1 Cup (250ml) Fresh Coriander, well rinsed and dried off with kitchen towel

- ½ Cup (125ml) Fresh cherry tomatoes, halved

- ¼ Cup (60ml) Fresh cucumber, sliced

- ¼ Cup (60ml) Raw carrot, sliced

- ¼ Cup (60ml) Raw green beans, julienned

- ¼ Cup (60ml) Mung bean sprouts

- 1 Tablespoon (15ml) Raw seed mix

- 1 Tablespoon (15ml) Raw cashew nuts, whole

Instructions:

1. On a serving plate, place the fresh coriander

2. Top with the Mung bean sprouts, cherry tomatoes, cucumber, carrot and green beans

3. Sprinkle over the raw seeds and cashew nuts and serve

Fresh Basil and Tomato Salad with Black Olives and Pine Nuts

The fresh basil is known for its anti-bacterial properties and has a unique flavor that pairs very well with the tomatoes and olives. Pine nuts are a great source of dietary fibre and protein, as well as essential fats and anti-oxidants.

Serves One

Ingredients:

- 1 Cup (250ml) Fresh basil leaves

- 1 Cup (250ml) Fresh cherry tomatoes, halved

- ½ Cup (125ml) Black olives, pitted

- ¼ Cup (60ml) Raw pine nuts

Instructions:

1. Place the fresh basil leaves on a serving plate

2. Top with the cherry tomatoes and olives

3. Sprinkle over the raw pine nuts and serve

Fresh Rocket (Arugula) Salad with Eggplant, Brazil Nuts and Avocado

Fresh rocket or arugula is high in essential minerals and dietary fibre; it also has a unique mustardy flavor that makes it a great base for any salad. Eggplant is a great source of vitamin B1 and manganese. The Brazil nuts bring the protein, selenium and some essential fats to this party, while the avocado provides its potassium content and additional healthy fat. In this case the eggplant must be cooked prior to preparing this salad, as it is not a vegetable that is particularly palatable when raw.

Serves One:

Ingredients:

- 1 Cup (250ml) Fresh rocket (arugula)

- 1 small eggplant, sliced

- 1 Tablespoon (15ml) Dried herb mix

- ½ Cup (125ml) Cherry tomatoes, halved

- ¼ Cup (60ml) Fresh cucumber, sliced

- ¼ Cup (60ml) Raw green beans, julienned

- ¼ Cup (60ml) Raw Brazil nuts, roughly chopped

- ¼ of a ripe avocado, sliced

Instructions to cook the eggplant:

1. Preheat the oven to 350 degrees (200 degrees Celsius)

2. Lay the eggplant slices on a non-stick baking sheet

3. Sprinkle with the mixed dried herbs

4. Cook for approximately 20 minutes, or until the egg plant slices begin to brown

5. Once cooked, transfer to a cooling rack to cool while you begin preparing the rest of the salad

Instructions to make the salad:

1. Place the fresh rocket (arugula) on a serving plate

2. Top with the cherry tomatoes, cucumber, green beans and cooled egg plant slices

3. Place the sliced avocado over the top

4. Lastly, sprinkle the chopped Brazil nuts over the top of the salad and serve

Carrot and Orange Salad with Almonds and Dates

Carrots are high in beta carotene and vitamin A; they contain essential anti-oxidants and are also a great source of dietary fibre. The combination of carrot and orange in this salad provides an abundance of vitamin C as well as a unique flavor.

Serves One

Ingredients:

- 1 Cup (250ml) Raw carrot, grated

- 1 medium sized orange, peeled and segmented

- ¼ Cup (60ml) Dates, chopped

- ¼ Cup (60ml) Raw almonds, roughly chopped

Instructions:

1. Place the grated carrot in a serving bowl and top with the orange segments

2. Add the dates and sprinkle over the chopped almonds

3. Toss together and serve

Apple, Pecan Nut and Cucumber Salad

Cucumber has a high liquid content so it's great for helping maintain hydration throughout the afternoon; it is also known to be a great addition to a diet that's keeping a healthy, glowing skin in mind. The low glycemic index of the apples will help you sustain your energy and stave off hunger until dinner time.

Serves One:

Ingredients

- 1 small red apple, cored and sliced

- 1 small green apple, cored and sliced

- ¼ Cup raw pecan nuts, roughly chopped

- ¼ Cup raw cucumber, sliced

- 1 tablespoon (15ml) lime juice

Instructions:

1. Place the apple slices on a serving plate

2. Drizzle over the lime juice in order to stop the apple from browning

3. Add the chopped pecan nuts and cucumber, serve

Raw Baby Spinach Salad with Zucchini, Tomatoes and Black Olives

Spinach is rich in essential minerals and protein; not to mention that everyone knows it for its high iron content, the absorption of which is greatly improved by the vitamin C in the tomatoes. Zucchini is a great source of dietary fibre and essential minerals and is one of those vegetables that can be enjoyed both raw and cooked.

Serves One

Ingredients:

- 1 Cup (250ml) Raw baby spinach

- 1 Cup (250ml) Raw zucchini, grated

- ½ Cup (125ml) Raw cherry tomatoes, halved

- ¼ Cup (60ml) Black olives, pitted and halved

- 1 Tablespoon (15ml) Extra Virgin olive oil

- 1 Tablespoon (15ml) Raw seed mix

Instructions:

1. Place the raw baby spinach onto a serving plate

2. Top with the grated zucchini and cherry tomatoes

3. Add the black olives

4. Sprinkle over the raw seed mix

5. Drizzle with the olive oil and serve

Butternut and Coriander Salad with Seeds and Pine Nuts

Butternut is high in dietary fibre, which makes it a great food choice when keeping a healthy heart in mind; it is also high in essential minerals and can be enjoyed both raw and cooked. The pairing of butternut and coriander, along with the pine nuts, makes this salad incredibly flavorful.

Serves One:

Ingredients:

- 1 Cup (250ml) Fresh coriander, well rinsed and dried with kitchen towel

- 1 Cup (250ml) Raw butternut, peeled and finely sliced

- ¼ Cup (60ml) Raw green beans, julienned

- ¼ Cup (60ml) Fresh Cherry tomatoes, halved

- ¼ Cup (60ml) Mung bean sprouts

- ½ Cup (125ml) Raw pine nuts

- 1 Tablespoon (15ml) Raw seed mix

- 1 Tablespoon (15ml) Sesame seed oil

Instructions:

1. Place the fresh coriander in a serving bowl

2. Top with the raw butternut, green beans, Mung bean sprouts and cherry tomatoes

3. Add the raw pine nuts and sprinkle the raw seeds over the top

4. Drizzle with the sesame seed oil and serve

Baby Spinach Salad with Sweet Peppers, Avocado and Pistachios

The combination of spinach and sweet peppers in this salad is another example of how the body's ability to absorb the high iron content of the spinach is boosted by pairing it with another vegetable that is high in vitamin C. The sweet peppers are a great source of vitamin C and add a variety of colour to this salad.

Serves One:

Ingredients:

- 1 Cup (250ml) Fresh baby spinach leaves

- ¼ Cup (60ml) Raw red sweet pepper, sliced

- ¼ Cup (60ml) Raw yellow sweet pepper, sliced

- ¼ Cup (60ml) Raw orange sweet pepper, sliced

- ¼ Cup (60ml) Raw green pepper, sliced

- ¼ Cup (60ml) Raw cherry tomatoes, halved

- ¼ Cup (60ml) Raw green beans, julienned

- ¼ Cup (60ml) Raw pistachios, roughly chopped

- ¼ of a ripe avocado

- 1 Tablespoon (15ml) Extra virgin avocado oil

Instructions:

- Place the baby spinach in a serving bowl

- Top with the mixed sweet peppers, tomatoes and green beans

- Add the raw pistachios

- Slice the avocado over the top of the salad and drizzle with the avocado oil, serve

Avocado Stuffed with Micro Herbs Salad, Raw Seeds and Pine Nuts

Micro herbs are the young seedlings of vegetables and herbs that are harvested within two weeks of germination; they are a trendy new addition to recipes and are believed to be far more mineral and nutrient rich than the vegetables and herbs that have come to full maturity. Nevertheless they are incredibly flavorful and make a great base for any salad, as this recipe will show.

Serves One:

Ingredients:

- 1 Ripe avocado, halved and pitted

- 1 Cup (250ml) Mixed micro herbs

- ¼ Cup (60ml) Cherry tomatoes, quartered

- ¼ Cup (60ml) Raw pine nuts

- 1 Tablespoon (15ml) Raw seed mix

- 1 Tablespoon (15ml) Extra virgin avocado oil

Instructions:

1. Place the avocado halves in a serving bowl

2. In a separate bowl, toss together the micro herb mix, cherry tomatoes, raw pine nuts and raw seeds

3. Stuff each avocado with the micro herb mix, you will have some mix spilling over into the bowl, but that's okay

4. Drizzle with the avocado oil and serve

Micro Herbs Salad with Papaya, Chili and Cashew Nuts

The combination of mustardy flavors from the micro herbs really compliments the sweetness of the papaya in this recipe. The cashew nuts add a really nice crunch and a hearty dose of protein. Chilies are known as immune boosters due to their high concentration of capsicum, and in this instance they also compliment the mustardy flavors of the micro herbs. The addition of cucumber helps quench the heat of the chili.

Serves One

Ingredients:

- 1 Cup (250ml) Mixed micro herbs

- 1 Cup (250ml) Diced fresh papaya

- ½ Cup (125ml) Fresh cucumber, finely sliced

- 1 Teaspoon (5ml) Fresh red chili, seeded and finely chopped

- ½ Cup (125ml) Raw cashew nuts, roughly chopped

- 1 Tablespoon (15ml) Coconut shavings

- 1 Tablespoon (15ml) Sesame seed oil

Instructions:

1. Place the micro herbs in a serving bowl

2. Top with the cucumber

3. Top with the papaya

4. Top with the cashew nuts

5. Sprinkle the chopped chili and coconut shavings over the top and toss together

6. Drizzle with the sesame seed oil and serve

Coriander, Pineapple and Brazil nut Salad

This salad is another spicy option that has a different take on flavor combinations. The pineapple goes very well with the coriander and the hint of chili adds the spicy kick, which is tamed by the sweetness of the pineapple. The Brazil nuts bring along some crunchy protein.

Serves One:

Ingredients:

- 1 Cup (250ml) Fresh coriander, well rinsed and dried off with kitchen towel

- 1 Cup (250ml) Fresh pineapple, diced

- 1 Teaspoon (5ml) Fresh red chili, seeded and finely chopped

- ½ Cup (125ml) Raw Brazil nuts, roughly chopped

- 1 Tablespoon (15ml) Coconut shavings

- 1 Tablespoon (15ml) Sesame seed oil

Instructions:

1. Place the fresh coriander leaves into a serving bowl

2. Top with the pineapple

3. Top with the Brazil nuts

4. Sprinkle over the chopped chili and toss together

5. Sprinkle over the coconut shavings

6. Drizzle with the sesame seed oil and serve

Fresh Rocket (Arugula) Salad with Pears, Pecans and Avocado

Here is yet another example of how one can get creative with flavor combinations while following a pegan diet. The mustardy flavor of the rocket (arugula) goes very well with the sweetness of the pears. The pecans add a protein crunch and the creaminess of the avocado brings all the flavors together in a comforting way. This recipe is best made with the brown Asian pears, but will work with the green pears if that's all you can get hold of.

Serves One

Ingredients:

- 1 Cup (250ml) Fresh rocket (arugula) leaves

- 1 large Asian pear, thinly sliced

- ½ Cup (125ml) Raw pecan nuts, roughly chopped

- ½ of a ripe avocado, sliced

- 1 Tablespoon (15ml) Raw seed mix

Instructions:

1. Place the rocket (arugula) leaves into a serving bowl

2. Top with the sliced pear

3. Top with the raw pecan nuts

4. Top with the sliced avocado

5. Sprinkle the raw seeds over the top of the salad and serve

Iceberg Lettuce Wraps with Carrot, Cucumber, Chili and Pistachios

The large leaves of an iceberg lettuce are a great alternative to a gluten and grain rich tortilla wrap. Lettuce has a high water content and when combined with the cucumber, this meal will really help you maintain hydration throughout a long hot afternoon. The chili compliments the buttery flavor of the protein rich pistachios and the carrots add a good dose of anti-oxidants.

Serves one (makes two wraps)

Ingredients:

- 2 large iceberg lettuce leaves

- ½ Cup (125ml) Raw carrot sticks

- ½ Cup (125ml) Raw cucumber sticks

- 1 Teaspoon (5ml) Fresh red chili, seeded and finely chopped

- ½ Cup (125ml) Raw pistachios, roughly chopped

- 1 Tablespoon (15ml) Sesame seed oil

Instructions:

1. Lay out each of the iceberg lettuce leaves onto a plate or kitchen counter work surface

2. Divide the carrot sticks between each lettuce leaf, placing them perpendicular to one edge of the lettuce leaf

3. Divide the cucumber sticks between each lettuce leaf in the same way as you did the carrot sticks

4. Divide the chopped chili between each lettuce leaf, sprinkling it over the carrot and cucumber

5. Divide the chopped pistachios between each lettuce leaf, sprinkling them over the other ingredients

6. Divide the sesame seed oil between each lettuce leaf, drizzling it over the other ingredients

7. Roll the lettuce leaf up, wrapping all the ingredients inside, serve

Iceberg Lettuce Wraps with Apple, Almonds and Avocado

The beauty of the iceberg lettuce wrap recipe is that it provides a base for many filling options. In this variation we have the combination of the apple's sweetness with the protein rich crunch of the almonds, which is comfortingly rounded off by the creaminess of the avocado. The coconut shavings add a little extra heart healthy fats as well as their unique complimentary flavor.

Serves one (makes two wraps)

Ingredients:

- 2 large iceberg lettuce leaves

- 1 small red apple, cored and finely sliced

- 1 small green apple, cored and finely sliced

- ½ Cup (125ml) Raw almonds, roughly chopped

- ½ of a ripe avocado, sliced

- 1 Tablespoon (15ml) Coconut shavings

- 1 Tablespoon (15ml) sesame seed oil

Instructions:

1. Lay out each of the iceberg lettuce leaves onto a plate or kitchen counter work surface

2. Divide the red apple slices between each lettuce leaf, placing them perpendicular to the edge of the leaf

3. Divide the green apple slices between each lettuce leaf, placing them on top of the red apple slices

4. Divide the chopped almonds between each leaf, sprinkling them over the apple slices

5. Divided the sliced avocado between each leaf, placing the slices on top of the other ingredients

6. Divide the coconut shavings between each leaf, sprinkling them over the other ingredients

7. Divide the sesame seed oil between each leaf, drizzling it over the other ingredients

8. Roll the lettuce leaf up, wrapping all the ingredients inside, serve

Iceberg Lettuce Wraps with Green Beans, Mung Bean Sprouts and Hazel nuts

Here is another example of the versatility of the iceberg lettuce wrap concept. In this recipe we have the crunchy sweetness of the green beans, combined with the earthy flavor of the Mung bean sprouts and the unique flavor of the protein rich hazel nuts.

Serves one (makes two wraps)

Ingredients:

- 2 large iceberg lettuce leaves

- ½ Cup (125ml) Raw green beans, julienned

- ½ Cup (125ml) Mung bean sprouts

- ½ Cup (125ml) Raw hazel nuts, roughly chopped

- 1 Tablespoon (15ml) Avocado oil

Instructions:

1. Lay out each of the iceberg lettuce leaves onto a plate or kitchen counter work surface

60

2. Divide the julienned green beans between each lettuce leaf, placing them perpendicular to the edge of the leaf

3. Divide the Mung bean sprouts between each lettuce leaf, placing them on top of the green beans

4. Divide the chopped hazel nuts between each lettuce leaf, sprinkling them over the other ingredients

5. Divide the avocado oil between each lettuce leaf, drizzling it over the other ingredients

6. Roll the lettuce leaf up, wrapping all the ingredients inside and serve.

Spinach Wraps with Cherry Tomatoes, Sweet Peppers, Pine nuts and Black Olives

Large spinach leaves also provide an alternative to the gluten, grain rich tortilla wrap and can be used in place of the iceberg lettuce leaves since they provide a different flavor base. In this Mediterranean inspired recipe, the combination of flavors goes very well together proving once again how a pegan diet can be both interesting and nutritious.

Serves one (makes two wraps)

Ingredients:

- 2 large spinach leaves

- ½ Cup (125ml) Small cherry tomatoes, halved

- 1 Tablespoon (15ml) Red sweet pepper, sliced

- 1 Tablespoon (15ml) Yellow sweet pepper, sliced

- 1 Tablespoon (15ml) Orange sweet pepper, sliced

- ¼ Cup (60ml) Black olives, pitted and halved

- ½ Cup (125ml) Raw pine nuts

- 1 Tablespoon (15ml) Extra virgin olive oil

Instructions:

1. Place the spinach leaves on a plate or kitchen work surface

2. Divide the cherry tomatoes between each spinach leaf, placing them on the leaf, perpendicular to the edge of the leaf

3. Divide the red sweet peppers between each leaf, placing them on top of the cherry tomatoes

4. Divide the rest of the sweet peppers as you did the red ones between each leaf, making sure that each spinach leave gets an equal amount of the varied colors of sweet peppers

5. Divide the black olives between each spinach leaf and place them on top of the of the other ingredients

6. Divide the pine nuts between each spinach leaf and sprinkle them over the other ingredients

7. Divide the olive oil between each spinach leaf and drizzle it over the other ingredients

8. Roll up each spinach leaf, wrapping all the ingredients inside.

Spinach Wraps with Strawberries, Pecan nuts, Coconut and Avocado

The flavor combination of the strawberries, pecan nuts and coconut along with the creaminess of the avocado give this spinach wrap variation a completely fresh take on the concept. The strawberries are high in anti-oxidants which help the body to absorb the abundance of iron that is provided by the raw spinach. This is another incredibly nutritious and creative meal that will see you through the afternoon.

Serves one (makes two wraps)

Ingredients:

- 2 large spinach leaves

- ½ Cup (125ml) Fresh strawberries, halved

- ½ Cup (125ml) Raw pecan nuts, roughly chopped

- ½ of a ripe avocado, sliced

- 1 Tablespoon (15ml) Coconut slices

- 1 Tablespoon (15ml) Avocado oil

Instructions:

1. Place the spinach leaves on a plate or a kitchen work surface

2. Divide the strawberries between each spinach leaf, placing them on the leaf perpendicular to the edge of the leaf

3. Divide the pecan nuts between each spinach leaf, placing them on top of the strawberries

4. Divide the avocado slices between each leaf, placing them on top of the other ingredients

5. Divide the coconut shavings between each leaf, sprinkling them over the other ingredients

6. Divide the avocado oil between each leaf, drizzling it over the other ingredients

7. Roll up the spinach leaves, wrapping all the ingredients inside, serve.

Spinach Wraps with Red Cabbage, Carrot, Grapes, Almonds and Avocado

Red cabbage is very high in dietary fibre, making this variation of the spinach wrap recipe another energy sustaining option to keep you going all afternoon. This is also another example of how interesting flavor combinations can come together to create a delicious healthy meal.

Serves one (makes two wraps)

Ingredients:

- 2 large spinach leaves

- ½ Cup (125ml) Raw red cabbage, shredded

- ½ Cup (125ml) Raw carrot, grated

- ¼ Cup (60ml) White grapes, halved

- ¼ Cup (60ml) Red grapes, halved

- ½ Cup (125ml) Raw almonds, roughly chopped

- ½ of a ripe avocado, sliced

- 1 Tablespoon (15ml) avocado oil

Instructions:

1. Place the spinach leaves on a plate or a kitchen work surface

2. Divide the shredded red cabbage between each spinach leaf, placing it on the leaf, perpendicular to the edge

3. Divide the grated carrot between the two spinach leaves, placing it on top of the shredded cabbage

4. Combine the two different colors of grapes and divide them between each spinach leaf, placing them on top of the other ingredients

5. Divide the raw almonds between each spinach leaf, sprinkling them over the other ingredients

6. Divide the sliced avocado between each spinach leaf, placing it over the other ingredients

7. Divide the avocado oil between each spinach leaf, drizzling it over the other ingredients

8. Roll up the spinach leaves, wrapping up all the ingredients in inside them and serve.

Dinners

Dinner is the last of our main meals that we have in the day and is just as important as the other two. A wholesome and nutritious dinner should keep you full throughout the fast of sleeping, but still be light enough so as not to cause any digestive discomfort that may disrupt your night's rest. One of the benefits of following the pegan diet is that your meals are high energy sustaining fibre but are light enough so as not to make you feel heavy and bloated while trying to sleep. The recipes in this section show how you can make a delicious and nutritious dinner every night.

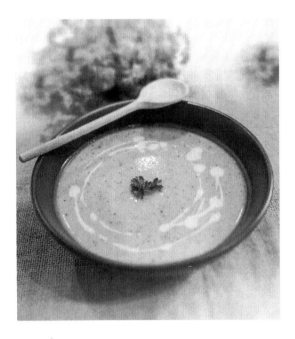

Pegan Ratatouille with Black Olives and Pine Nuts

What makes this fresh take on a classic recipe pegan is that it is raw. This recipe also shows how the right combination of flavors can still produce a tasty and nutritious meal without you having to cook all the ingredients. This dinner will definitely fill you up for the night, while providing a well-rounded source of vitamins, essential minerals and protein.

Serves One

Ingredients:

- 1 Cup (250ml) Fresh cherry tomatoes, halved

- 1 Cup (250ml) Raw zucchini, thinly sliced

- 1 small red onion, finely chopped

- 1 teaspoon (5ml) fresh garlic, finely chopped

- ¼ Cup (60ml) Fresh basil leaves, finely chopped

- ½ Cup (125ml) Black olives, pitted and halved

- ½ Cup (125ml) Raw pine nuts

- 2 Tablespoons (30ml) Extra virgin olive oil

Instructions:

1. Place the cherry tomatoes in to a serving bowl

2. Add the chopped onion, garlic and fresh basil

3. Add the black olives

4. Add the pine nuts

5. Drizzle over the olive oil and toss together

6. Allow to stand in the refrigerator for about one hour so that the flavors can marinate together before serving.

Raw Butternut Curry with Cashew Nuts and Coconut

You don't have to cook in order to enjoy a good curry. This recipe will show how you can enjoy all the flavors of a curry without standing over a hot stove for hours. Butternut is usually a vegetable that is eaten cooked, but this is another recipe that shows how it can be really delicious raw. The cashew nuts give you a solid protein source as well as healthy fats that will be slowly digested, keeping you full all night.

Serves One

Ingredients:

- 1 Cup (250ml) Raw butternut, peeled and finely sliced

- ½ Cup (125ml) Raw cashew nuts, roughly chopped

- 1 Tablespoon (15ml) Coconut shavings

- 1 teaspoon (5ml) Fresh red chili, seeded and finely chopped

- 1 teaspoon (5ml) Fresh ginger root, finely chopped

- 1 teaspoon (5ml) Fresh garlic, finely chopped

- 1 teaspoon (5ml) Fresh coriander, finely chopped

- 2 tablespoons (30ml) Extra virgin coconut oil

Instructions:

1. Place the finely sliced butternut into a serving bowl

2. Add the chopped ginger, garlic, chili and coriander

3. Add the cashew nuts and the coconut shavings

4. Drizzle over the coconut oil and toss all together

5. Allow to stand in the refrigerator for about an hour so that the flavors can marinate together before serving

Stuffed Gem Squash with Brazil nuts, Cabbage and Tomatoes

This is one recipe that does require a little cooking as gem squash seem to be more palatable when cooked, but it is only the gem squash that will require cooking. The combination of high fibre foods in this recipe make it another great option when choosing what to have for dinner as it will be slowly digested without weighing you down. In this instance we will have to imagine that our ancestors had a microwave oven.

Serves One:

Ingredients:

- 1 medium sized gem squash or any other kind of squash that is roughly the size of a soft ball

- 1 Cup (250ml) Red cabbage, shredded

- 1 Cup (250ml) Fresh cherry tomatoes, halved

- ½ Cup (125ml) Raw Brazil nuts, roughly chopped

- 1 teaspoon (5ml) Fresh garlic, finely chopped

- 1 teaspoon (5ml) Fresh basil leaves, finely chopped

- 2 Tablespoons (30ml) Black olives, pitted and finely chopped

- 2 Tablespoons (30ml) Extra virgin olive oil

- 1 Tablespoon (15ml) Raw pumpkin seeds

Instructions to cook the gem squash:

1. Cut the gem squash in half and remove the seeds

2. Place in the microwave on 100% power for approximately 5 minutes, you want the gem squash to be cooked, but still retaining its shape

3. Set aside to cool while you prepare the stuffing

Instructions to make the stuffing:

1. Place the shredded cabbage in a bowl

2. Add the chopped garlic, fresh basil leaves, cherry tomatoes, black olives, Brazil nuts and olive oil

3. Toss together and allow to sit in the refrigerator for approximately one hour so that the flavors can marinate together

Instructions to assemble the stuffed gem squash:

1. Place the cooked gem squash halves in a serving bowl, it will be easier to use a bowl rather than a plate because this way you can still catch any over-flowing stuffing

2. Divide the now well marinated stuffing between the two gem squash halves

3. Divide the raw pumpkin seeds between the now stuffed gem squash halves, sprinkling them over the top and serve.

Tomatoes stuffed with Baby Spinach, Pine Nuts and Black Olives

Tomatoes are not only incredibly nutritious, but they are also very versatile as they are easily enjoyed both cooked and raw. This recipe once again shows how a dish that would usually be served cooked can be enjoyed raw and still be just as flavorful and satisfying.

Serves One

Ingredients:

- 2 large tomatoes

- 1 Cup (250ml) Baby spinach leaves

- ½ Cup (125ml) Raw pine nuts

- ¼ Cup (60ml) Black olives, pitted and roughly chopped

- 1 teaspoon (5ml) fresh garlic, finely chopped

- 1 teaspoon (5ml) fresh basil leaves, finely chopped

- 2 Tablespoons (30ml) extra virgin olive oil

Instructions:

1. Slice the top off of each tomato and scoop out the insides into a bowl so that you are left with a tomato shell.

2. Place the tomato shells upside down on a plate so that any remaining juice can drain out of them

3. Roughly chop up the tomato flesh that you have scooped out of the shells

4. To the bowl that contains the tomato flesh, add the baby spinach leaves, chopped garlic, basil leaves, black olives and pine nuts

5. Drizzle over the olive oil and toss together

6. Allow the stuffing mixture to sit in the refrigerator for about one hour so that all the flavors can marinate together

7. Once the stuffing has marinated, place the tomato shells in a serving bowl and divide the stuffing between each tomato shell, making sure you fill them to the brim

8. Drizzle over a little extra virgin olive oil and serve

Avocados Stuffed with Apple and Walnuts

Avocados are incredibly nutritious and their high potassium and healthy fat content make them a great base for a wholesome meal. The high dietary fibre content of the apples will keep you full and any hunger pangs very much at bay all night. The walnuts provide a healthy dose of essential minerals and are a great source of protein. This dish is another interesting flavor combination that proves how creative one can be while following the pegan lifestyle.

Serves One

Ingredients:

- 1 medium sized ripe avocado, halved and pitted

- 1 small red apple, cored and finely chopped

- 1 small green apple, cored and finely chopped

- ½ Cup (125ml) Raw walnuts, roughly chopped

- 2 Tablespoons (30ml) Avocado oil

- 1 Tablespoon (15ml) Coconut shavings

Instructions:

1. In a bowl mix together the apples, walnuts and avocado oil

2. Place the avocado halves in a serving bowl

3. Stuff the avocados with the apple and walnut mixture, it's okay if some of the stuffing spills over into the bowl

4. Sprinkle the coconut shavings over the top and serve

Avocados Stuffed with Strawberries, Pecan nuts and Rocket (Arugula)

This recipe is a different take on the flavor combinations of one the previous spinach wrap recipes and also shows the versatility of the avocado. The sweetness of the strawberries combined with the mustardy flavor of the rocket (arugula) goes incredibly well with the earthy unique flavor of the pecan nuts; and all comes together nicely with the creaminess of the avocado.

Serves One

Ingredients:

- 1 medium sized ripe avocado, halved and pitted

- 1 Cup (250ml) Fresh strawberries, quartered

- ½ Cup (125ml) Raw pecan nuts, roughly chopped

- ½ Cup (125ml) Fresh rocket (arugula) leaves, finely chopped

- 2 Tablespoons (30ml) Avocado oil

- 1 Tablespoon (15ml) Raw seed mix

- 1 Tablespoon (15ml) Coconut shavings

Instructions:

1. In a bowl, combine the strawberries, pecan nuts, fresh rocket (arugula), raw seed mix and the avocado oil

2. Toss together

3. Place the avocado halves in a serving bowl

4. Stuff the avocado halves with the strawberry mixture, it's okay if some stuffing spills over into the bowl

5. Sprinkle over the coconut shavings and serve

Tomatoes Stuffed with Avocado, Pistachios, Micro Herbs and Bean Sprouts

This recipe is another take on the previous stuffed tomato recipe and provides a very wholesome and tasty dinner. Again we have an example of how creative flavor combinations can come together in order to keep every meal interesting as well as satisfying.

Serves One:

Ingredients:

- Two large tomatoes

- ½ of a ripe avocado, sliced

- ½ Cup (125ml) Mixed micro herbs

- ½ Cup (125ml) Bean sprouts

- ½ Cup (125ml) Raw pistachios, roughly chopped

- 2 tablespoons (30ml) Extra virgin olive oil

Instructions:

1. Slice the top off of each tomato and scoop out the insides into a bowl so that you are left with a tomato shell.

2. Place the tomato shells upside down on a plate so that any remaining juice can drain out of them

3. Roughly chop up the tomato flesh that you have scooped out of the shells

4. To the bowl that contains the tomato flesh, add the micro herbs, bean sprouts, avocado and pistachios

5. Drizzle over the olive oil and toss together

6. Allow the stuffing mixture to sit in the refrigerator for about one hour so that all the flavors can marinate together

7. Once the stuffing has marinated, place the tomato shells in a serving bowl and divide the stuffing between each tomato shell, making sure you fill them to the brim

8. Drizzle over a little extra olive oil and serve

Zucchini Stuffed with Micro Herbs, Avocado and Pine Nuts

When weighing up the pros and cons of eating your vegetables raw, this recipe will show how a zucchini can be a little more versatile when enjoyed as such. This recipe is a little finicky to prepare, but if you manage to find large enough zucchinis then you shouldn't have too much trouble. The interesting flavor combinations will get you excited about taking the time to prepare this meal and the high fibre content of the raw zucchini will be sure to keep your hunger satisfied all night.

Serves One:

Ingredients:

- 2 large raw zucchinis, as large as you can find that will still be easy to finish as a meal

- ½ Cup (125ml) Mixed micro herbs

- ½ Cup (125ml) Raw pine nuts

- ½ of a ripe avocado, diced

- 2 Tablespoon (30ml) Extra virgin olive oil

- 1 Tablespoon (15ml) Raw seed mix

Instructions:

1. Cut the zucchinis in half an scoop out the flesh using a teaspoon

2. Chop the zucchini flesh and place it in a bowl

3. To the bowl that contains the zucchini flesh, add the micro herbs, pine nuts and avocado.

4. Toss together with the olive oil

5. Place the zucchini shells on serving plate

6. Stuff the zucchini shells with the micro herb mixture

7. Sprinkle the raw seed mix over the top

8. Drizzle over a little extra virgin olive oil and serve

Natural Detox Carrot Soup

With this amazing raw food recipe, you can boost your immune system with massive amounts of vitamins C and A. Ginger is great for digestive problems and acts as a natural anti-inflammatory.

Serves: 2

Ingredients:

- 4 large carrots (peeled unless organic) and chopped
- Juice of 1 orange
- 1 mango, peeled, pitted and chopped
- 2 inches of ginger
- 1 big onion
- 1 red bell pepper
- 2 garlic cloves
- ½ cup cilantro, chopped
- 2 cups coconut milk
- 1 tablespoon olive oil
- ¼ cup sunflower seeds
- Himalayan/sea salt to taste

Instructions:

1. Place all the ingredients (except cilantro, sunflower seeds and oil) in a blender. Blend until smooth and creamy.
2. Add a pinch of Himalayan salt to taste. Sprinkle some olive oil, cilantro and sunflower seeds over the soup.
3. Enjoy!

Spicy Exotic Soup or Smoothie

Greens are super alkalizing so use them in your pegan smoothies. You can use your blender to create nutrient-packed, dense smoothies almost like soups or vegetable creams. They are quick and easy to prepare and a fantastic way of eating in the summer. In the winter, you may heat them up slightly, it's up to you!

Serves: 2

Ingredients:

- 1 cup coconut milk
- 2 cups filtered water (preferably alkaline water)
- 1/4 cup cilantro
- 1/2 cup spinach leaves
- 1 zucchini
- 2 garlic cloves
- ½ cup of radish
- 1/4 cup of cashews (soaked in water for a few hours)
- 1/2 tsp. turmeric powder
- 1/4 tsp black pepper (real game changer as it helps your body get all the anti-inflammatory benefits that turmeric powder offers)
- 1/4 Himalayan salt

- 1 tablespoon organic, cold-pressed, virgin olive oil

Instructions:

1. Blend well, squeeze some fresh lime or lemon juice into the mixture, and enjoy!
2. Serve cold or slightly heated (but keep it raw).

Raw Veggie Noodles

Easy, tasty and delicious!

Serves: 2

Ingredients:

- 4 carrots
- 2 cucumbers
- 1 zucchini
- 1 tablespoon of coconut oil
- A few cilantro leaves
- ½ cup radish
- ¼ cup of dried fruit of your choice
- 1 avocado, peeled, pitted and sliced
- Organic, cold-pressed virgin olive oil
- Apple cider vinegar or lemon juice
- Himalaya salt

Instructions:

1. First, place carrots, cucumbers and zucchini through a spiralizer to create a noodle-like shape.
2. Place carrots, cucumbers, dried fruits and avocado in a salad bowl.

3. Now, stir-fry the zucchini noodles in coconut oil using extremely low heat. You just want zucchini to soften up a bit and absorb the coconut flavor.
4. When done, add zucchini into the salad bowl and mix well with other ingredients.
5. Sprinkle some olive oil, lemon juice or vinegar over the salad.
6. Season with Himalayan salt and garnish with cilantro leaves.
7. Enjoy!

Summer Party

Serves: 4

Ingredients:

- 1 red organic beetroot, peeled and sliced
- 6 whole radishes, sliced
- 1 beetroot, peeled and sliced
- 1/2 of a red onion, peeled and sliced
- 2 small zucchini, sliced and steamed to soften up
- 1 small kohlrabi, sliced
- 1 red pepper, deseeded and sliced
- ¼ cup of sunflower seeds

Dressing:
- 2 tablespoons of olive oil (extra virgin)
- 2 teaspoons of fresh oregano, chopped
- 1 clove of garlic, peeled and finely chopped
- 1 teaspoon of organic maple syrup
- 1 tablespoon of fresh parsley leaves, chopped
- Fresh juice of 1 lemon
- Himalayan salt to taste

Instructions:

1. To make the dressing, whisk some olive oil with 1 clove of chopped garlic and maple syrup.
2. Add lemon juice, sea salt, parsley, and oregano.
3. Whisk again to combine.
4. Set aside in a fridge while you are preparing the salad.
5. Mix the sliced veggies in a big bowl.
6. Add some sunflower seeds and drizzle the salad dressing on top to serve the salad.

Papaya Salad

Ingredients: (2-3 servings)

- 1 cup mixed fresh lettuce leaves
- 1 small green papaya, julienned
- ½ cup whole radish, sliced
- 2 carrots, peeled and spiralized (or sliced thinly)
- 1/ 2 cup of raw cashew nuts
- 1 cup cherry tomatoes, halved

For the Chili Spicy Dressing:

- 1 tablespoon of raw coconut vinegar
- 1 tablespoon of cane sugar or maple syrup
- 1 red long chili, seeded and finely chopped
- Juice of 2 limes
- 1 small clove of garlic, peeled and minced

Instructions:

1. Whisk all the dressing ingredients in a small bowl. Set aside in a fridge to cool.
2. In the meantime, prepare the salad by tossing all the salad ingredients together in a salad bowl.
3. Now mix the salad with the dressing so that all ingredients are equally covered.
4. Serve with some lemon wedges. Enjoy!

Easy Chia Snack

Great as a natural, after-dinner treat or a snack during the day!

Serves: 1-2

Ingredients:

- 2 tbsp. chia seeds
- 1 tbsp. coconut milk powder
- 1 tbsp. maple syrup

Toppings:

- Half a cup of blueberries
- 1 pear spiralized

Preparation:

1. Grind the chia seeds in a blender with a grinder attachment like if you wanted to grind coffee beans.
2. Add the coconut milk powder and water and heat to boiling point. You can omit this step if you want it to be a cold pudding.
3. Whisk the ground chia seeds into the liquid. Whisk again after a few minutes. Leave the mixture until it thickens and serve with a drizzle of maple syrup. Top it with blueberries and a spiralized pear for a delicious breakfast or in-between meals during the day.

Raw Thai Salad with Spiralized Zucchini

Serves: 2

Ingredients:

- 2 medium zucchini, noodles
- 2 carrots, noodle
- ½ cup green onions (shallots), finely chopped
- 1 medium bell pepper, julienned
- 1 cup finely chopped red cabbage
- 1 green apple julienned
- 1 cup of cauliflower cut into small pieces

Put everything in a large bowl.

Sauce:

- 4 dates soaked in warm water for about thirty minutes (you can substitute dried tomatoes)
- ½ cup butter nuts (almonds, cashews, or even peanuts)
- 3 tbsp. of agave nectar
- 3 tbsp. tamari (soy sauce)

- Juice of one lime
- 1 tsp chili pepper or chili sauce to taste. Garnish with spiralized zucchini.

Preparation:

1. Place ingredients in a food processor and blend until it sounds sauce. If too thick, add a little water.
2. Pour over vegetables. Mix well.

Spiralized Carrot and Cucumber Roast

Serves: 2

Ingredients:

- 5 cucumbers, small or medium, peeled, cut lengthwise into 2
- 6 carrots, peeled, spiralized
- 2 tbsp. extra virgin olive oil
- 1 head garlic, cloves in defeat, peeled
- To taste sea salt and freshly ground pepper

Preparation:

1. In a shallow baking dish, pour the oil to coat the bottom. Add the garlic and also season with sea salt and pepper. Add in the vegetables and coat well by stirring in the seasoned oil. Vegetables should be placed in a single layer and not stacked so that they are well roasted. Pour a little olive oil over the vegetables.

2. Preheat the oven to 400 °F (200 Celsius) and cook the vegetables for 15 minutes. Vegetables should be tender and golden.

Root Salad with a Lychee Dressing

Serves: 2

Ingredients:

• 1 cup lychee water

• 1 cup almond nuts

• 2 beetroots spiralized on a regular setting

• 5 cherry tomatoes diced

Preparation:

1. Blend lychee water and almond nuts in a blender until smooth.

2. Then, pour it over the veggies.

3. Garnish with chopped tomatoes.

Leek and Mushroom Soup

Serves: 2

Ingredients:

- 1 tbsp. olive oil
- 2 leeks, chopped
- 2 cloves garlic, minced
- 1 ½ lb. mushrooms   (nearly 3 cups)
- 1 qt. low-sodium vegetable broth (4 cups)
- ¼ cup chopped cilantro

Carrots and parsnip topping:

- 1 cup of parsnips, sliced, blanched for 2 minutes
- 2 carrots, peeled and sliced

Preparation:

1. Heat oil in large saucepan over a medium heat. Add leeks and garlic and sauté for 5 to 7 minutes or until the leeks are soft. Add mushrooms and cook 5 minutes or until most of the liquid has evaporated.

2. Add the vegetable broth, cilantro and simmer for 5 minutes. Reduce heat to medium-low and simmer for 15 more minutes.

3. Purée the soup in batches until smooth.

4. Garnish the soup with blanched parsnips and carrots.

Easy Ginger and Almond Soup

This soup requires no cooking and can be eaten hot or cold. Adding very thinly sliced radishes will add a zing to this delicious raw soup.

Serves: 2

Ingredients:

- A small piece of fresh ginger
- ½ clove of garlic, peeled and chopped
- Handful of almonds, crushed
- 4 cups of hot water
- A small piece of fresh turmeric
- Handful of fresh parsley
- 3 radishes, sliced

Preparation:

1. Place all the ingredients in a blender and well mix until you obtain a smooth mixture.
2. If you want a hot soup, use hot water instead. Garnish with spiralized radishes.

Beet Salad with a Coconut Dressing

Serves: 2

Ingredients:

•1 cup young coconut water

•5 plum tomatoes, sliced

•1 cup macadamia nuts

•2 beets, sliced

•5 rosemary leaves

Preparation:

1. In a blender blitz the macadamia nuts and coconut water until smooth.

2. Add the beets on top and garnish with rosemary and sliced plum tomatoes.

Spicy Pepper Salad

Serves: 1-2

Ingredients:

For the dressing:

•2 yellow and red bell peppers, diced

•1 tbsp. chili powder

•A pinch of paprika powder

•3 tbsp. lime juice

•Sea salt to taste

For the salad:

•3 cups spinach leaves

•1 red bell pepper, spiralized

Preparation:

1. Combine all the ingredients in a high speed blender and blitz until smooth.

2. Place the greens in a salad bowl then scatter the peppers.

3. Lastly, liberally drizzle on the dressing and serve.

Comfort Mushroom Soup

Serves: 1-2

Ingredients:

- 1 tbsp. olive oil
- 2 leeks, chopped
- 2 cloves garlic, minced
- 1 ½ lb. mushrooms
- 1 qt. low-sodium vegetable broth
- 3 fresh thyme strings
- ¼ cup chopped cilantro

Carrots and parsnip topping:

- 1 cup of spiralized carrots and parsnips, blanched for 2 minutes

Preparation:

1. Heat oil in large saucepan over a medium heat. Add leeks and garlic and sauté for 5 to 7 minutes or until the leeks are soft. Add mushrooms and cook 5 minutes or until most of the liquid has evaporated.

2. Add the broth, thyme, cilantro and simmer. Reduce the heat to medium-low and simmer for a further 15 minutes.

3. Purée the soup in batches until smooth and season to your taste.

4. Garnish the soup with spiralized blanched carrots and parsnips.

Fresh Fruit Skewers with Vegan Coconut Yoghurt Dip

Fruit is an incredibly healthy and nutritious snack alternative to sugar laden sweets. The natural sugars in fruits are slowly released and therefore help in maintaining blood sugar without giving you that horrible spike that comes from refined sugar. These skewers are easy to prepare in advance and make a great addition to any lunch box or picnic basket. The coconut yoghurt dip not only adds protein, but also a little extra comfort to this snack combination.

Makes approximately 10 Skewers

Ingredients to make the fruit skewers:

- 1 medium sized fresh papaya, peeled, pitted and cubed

- 1 medium sized fresh pineapple, peeled and cubed

- 1 Cup fresh white seedless grapes, whole

- 1 Cup fresh black seedless grapes, whole

- 1 Cup whole dates

Instructions to make the fruit skewers:

1. Using either wooden or bamboo skewer sticks place the fruit pieces on the skewer sticks, alternating with a single piece of the different fruits at a time. For example, 1 piece papaya, 1 piece pineapple, 1 white grape, 1 date, 1 red grape.

2. Continue until the skewer is full and then begin the next one

3. Once all the fruit is has been skewered, place the fruit skewers on a serving plate or into a tub for refrigeration.

Ingredients to make the vegan yoghurt dip:

- 1 Cup vegan coconut yogurt (or other vegan yoghurt of your choice)

- ¼ Cup Coconut Cream

- 1 Teaspoon Vanilla Essence

- ½ Teaspoon Ground Cinnamon

- 1 Teaspoon Raw Cocoa Powder

- 1 Tablespoon Desiccated Coconut

- 1 Tablespoon Dried Berry mix

Instructions to make the vegan yoghurt dip:

1. Place the yoghurt and coconut cream into a mixing bowl

2. Add the vanilla essence, ground cinnamon and raw cocoa powder

3. Whisk well

4. Stir in the desiccated coconut and the dried berry mix

5. If you are serving the fruit skewers at home then place the yoghurt dip into a serving dish. If you are taking the skewers to go, then place the yoghurt dip into a take away container. Both the yoghurt dip and the fruit skewers are best kept refrigerated, so if you are taking them in your lunch box or to a picnic, ensure that they are in a cooler bag.

Fresh Basil, Cherry Tomato Salad

There is just something amazing about the flavor combination of tomato and basil. This salad is a tasty, nutritious reason to take a break from your desk.

Serves One

Ingredients:

- ½ Cup Fresh Basil leaves

- ½ Cup Cherry tomatoes, halved

- 1 Tablespoon Raw Pine nuts

- 2 Teaspoons Organic Extra Virgin Olive Oil

Instructions:

1. In a serving bowl, or take away tub, place the fresh basil leaves

2. Add the halved cherry tomatoes

3. Top with the raw pine nuts

4. Just before serving drizzle with the olive oil and toss well. Salt and pepper can be added to taste.

Red Cabbage, Cucumber, and Pomegranate Salad with Pomegranate dressing

Serves One:

Ingredients for the salad:

- 1 Cup Raw Red Cabbage, shredded

- ½ Cup Cucumber Slices

- ¼ Cup Pomegranate Seeds

- 1 Tablespoon Raw Seed Mix

Ingredients for the dressing:

- ¼ Cup Fresh pomegranate juice

- 1 Tablespoon Extra Virgin Coconut Oil

- ¼ Teaspoon Organic Ground Sea Salt

- ¼ Teaspoon Ground Black Pepper

Instructions to make the salad:

1. In a serving bowl, or a take away tub, place the raw red cabbage

2. Add the cucumber

3. Add the pomegranate seeds

4. Add the raw seed mix

Instructions to make the dressing:

1. In a large mixing jug combine the pomegranate juice, coconut oil, salt and pepper.

2. Whisk well

3. Just before serving, pour the dressing over the salad and toss together

Homemade Trail Mix

Trail mix is another great on-the-go snack option, but very often the pre-packed versions that we buy in the supermarkets contain unnecessary additives and preservatives. By mixing your own trail mix, using organic, raw ingredients you are ensuring that you get a healthy, energy-boosting snack that you can trust. This recipe includes dried berry mix and raw cocoa nibs, making it a great source of anti-oxidants as well.

Makes approximately 4 ¼ Cup

Ingredients:

- 4 Tablespoons   Raw Cashew Nuts, whole

- 4 Tablespoons Raw Brazil Nuts, Whole

- 4 Tablespoons Raw Seed mix

- 4 Tablespoons Dried Berry Mix

- 4 Tablespoons Coconut Flakes

- 4 Tablespoons Raw Cocoa Nibs

- 4 Tablespoons Dried Mango Pieces

- 4 Tablespoons Dried Apple Pieces

Instructions:

1. Place all the ingredients into a large mixing bowl and toss together well

2. Using a ¼ cup measuring cup, divide the trail mix into portions

3. You can either place each portion in a small sandwich bag, or a small take away tub.

4. If you choose not to pre-portion out the entire mix, then you can store it in an airtight glass jar.

BONUS-Healing Pegan Smoothie Recipes

Easy Green Smoothie

Serves 1-2

Ingredients

- 1 tablespoon olive oil
- ½ cup of apple juice
- ½ cup of broccoli
- ½ cup of artichokes
- ½ cup of kale
- ½ cup of arugula
- 1 pear
- Dash of salt

Directions

1. Cook the broccoli so it is soft.
2. Buy artichokes in a glass container.

3. Add olive oil, apple juice, broccoli, and artichokes to the blender and mix on low to medium.
4. Then pull the kale leaves from the kale stems.
5. Cut the pear in half and peel away the skin.
6. Then cut away the core and stem.
7. Put pear meat and the kale into the blender and mix on low to medium.
8. Put the dash of salt in with the ingredients.
9. Mix all the ingredients until they are all in small pieces and the liquid is smooth to drink. Taste and adjust if you need to. When the smoothie is ready pour the smoothie into a glass with a straw.

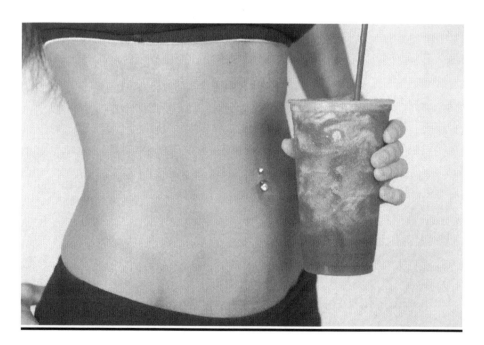

Soothing Lavender Pegan Smoothie

Serves 1-2

Ingredients

- 1 teaspoon of culinary lavender
- 2 cups of water
- 2 sprigs of mint
- ½ cucumber
- ½ cup of Strawberries
- 1 teaspoon Spirulina

Directions

1. In a large glass jug add the teaspoon of culinary lavender and the 2 cups of water.
2. Put the two sprigs of mint into the jug.
3. Put in the refrigerator for two hours and take out the sprig of mint.
4. Then keep the lavender mixture in the refrigerator for three more hours.
5. Then strain the lavender from the water.
6. Add lavender water to the blender.

7. Peel the cucumber and measure out ½ cup of cucumber meat and put it in the blender. Cut the green leaves off of the strawberries.

8. Also add the strawberries and Spirulina to the blender.

9. Mix all the ingredients together until smooth and well blended.

10. Taste and adjust if you need to.

11. Serve the smoothie in a glass cold with a straw to drink.

Vanilla Smoothie

Serves 1-2

Ingredients

- 1 natural vanilla bean
- ½ cup of cashew milk
- ½ banana
- 2 tablespoons nutritional yeast
- ½ cup of kale

Directions

1. Take the vanilla bean and press it flat with your fingers.
2. Then take a knife and gently split the vanilla bean open and scoop out the fresh vanilla specs with a spoon.
3. Pour the cashew milk into the blender.
4. Peel the banana and put the banana into the blender.
5. Then put the vanilla and the nutritional yeast in the mix.
6. Also separate the kale leaves from the stems and add the kale to the blender as well. Turn the speed on low and gradually use medium in order to blend all the ingredients together.

7. Blend the mix well so everything is pureed. When smoothie is at desired flavor, pour the smoothie into a glass and serve with a straw.

Cinnamon Smoothie

Serves 1-2

Ingredients

- 2 teaspoons of cinnamon
- ½ cup of almond milk
- 1 apple
- ½ cup of broccoli
- 1 teaspoon barley grass

Directions

1. Cook the broccoli just until it is soft.
2. Pour the almond milk in the blender.
3. Add the ingredients of cinnamon and broccoli along with the barley grass.
4. You can buy fresh cinnamon sticks and grate the cinnamon sticks with a grater until you have enough to fill two teaspoons.
5. Take the peel off of the apple and remove the seed, stem, if it has one, and the core.
6. Put the apple meat into the blender.
7. Turn the blender speed to low and gradually raise to medium.

8. Mix all of the ingredients together until well blended.
9. Taste your smoothie and adjust if you need to by adding a small amount of one or more of the ingredients.
10. When you have your desired flavor, pour the smoothie into a glass and serve with a straw.

Ashwagandha Herbal Coconut Smoothie

Serves 1-2

Ingredients

- 1 teaspoon of Ashwagandha powder
- ½ coconut milk
- 1 frozen banana
- 1 apple
- 3 dates
- ½ cup of blueberries
- ½ teaspoon of lime juice

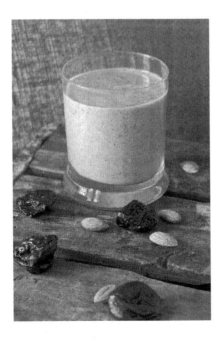

Directions

1. Warm up the coconut milk in a stainless steel pan on a medium heat.
2. Add the Ashwagandha powder to the warm milk and stir while it is on a low heat.
3. Put the mixture in the refrigerator to cool.
4. You can make the Ashwagandha and coconut mix the night before.
5. Peel the apple and remove the stem and core.
6. Remove the pits from the dates and put the dates in the blender.
7. Add also the lime and apple meat.
8. Mix all the ingredients on a low to medium speed.
9. Mix them well so that all the flavors mix together.
10. Try the smoothie and add a little of one or more ingredients if it needs it.
11. When the smoothie is ready pour the smoothie into a glass with a straw.

Grape Smoothie

Serves 1-2

Ingredients

- 1 cup of seedless grapes
- 1 pear
- ½ cup of cranberry juice
- ½ cup of broccoli

Directions

1. Put the grapes into the blender.
2. Take the skin off of the pear and take out the core and the stem.
3. Put the pear meat into the blender along with the cranberry juice.
4. Cook the broccoli just until soft, then cool the broccoli in the refrigerator.
5. Put the broccoli in the blender with the other ingredients.
6. Put the speed on low to medium and mix together the ingredients until they are well blended.
7. Try the smoothie and add a small amount of one or more of the ingredients.

8. When the smoothie is ready pour the well-blended mix in a glass and serve with a straw.

Your Free Gift

Don't forget to download your free complimentary recipe eBook:

www.bitly.com/karenfreegift

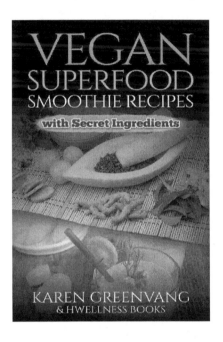

If you have any problems with your download, email me at: karenveganbooks@gmail.com

Conclusion

Thank you for reading!

I hope that with so many vegan recipes you will be motivated and inspired to start and/or continue your journey towards meaningful veganism, vibrant health and total wellbeing.

Remember, the beauty of incorporating nutritious vegan foods into your daily diet is that you are making simple, yet sustainable changes that will work for your wellness long-term. Not to mention your spiritual wellness and taking care of the environment.

If you enjoyed my book, it would be greatly appreciated if you left a review so others can receive the same benefits you have. Your review can help other people take this important step to take care of their health and inspire them to start a new chapter in their lives.

At the same time, <u>you can help me serve you and all my other readers</u> even more through my next vegan-friendly recipe books that I am committed to publishing on a regular basis.

I'd be thrilled to hear from you. I would love to know your favorite recipe(s).

Don't be shy, post a comment on Amazon! Your comments are really important to me.

→ Questions about this book? Email me at: karenveganbooks@gmail.com

Thank You for your time,

Love & Light,

Until next time-

Karen Vegan Greenvang

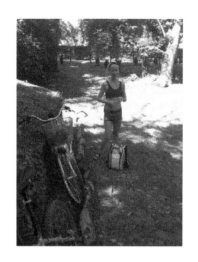

More Vegan Books by Karen

Available in kindle and paperback in all Amazon stores.

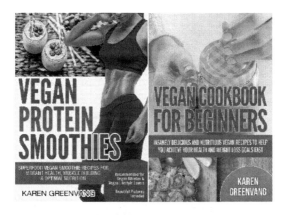

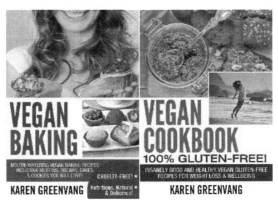

You will find more at:

www.amazon.com/author/karengreenvang

You can also search for "Karen Greenvang" in your local Amazon store.

59345525R00076

Made in the USA
Lexington, KY
02 January 2017